Fit Over 40 Challenge

Six Weeks to Lose Fat,
Build Muscle and Feel
20 Years Younger

David McGarry

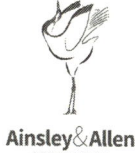

Ainsley&Allen
PUBLISHING

Copyright © 2017 by Ainsley & Allen Publishing.

All rights reserved. No part of this publication may be reproduced, distributed or transmitted in any form or by any means, including photocopying, recording, or other electronic or mechanical methods, without the prior written permission of the publisher, except in the case of brief quotations embodied in critical reviews and certain other noncommercial uses permitted by copyright law. For permission requests, write to the publisher, addressed "Attention: Permissions Coordinator," at the address below.

Ainsley & Allen Publishing LLC
2035 Sunset Lake Road
Newark, DE 19702
www.ainsleyallenpublishing.com

Fit Over 40 Challenge—1st ed.

ISBN-13: 978-0-9975855-5-1
ISBN-10: 0997585552

Dedication

My Dad

Dad, I can't believe that it has been ten years since I last heard your voice that Saturday morning in May. You were such an amazing dad and person. I know everything happens for a reason and I hope that out of this tragedy and our loss this book will help inspire and motivate one person to change their life.

My Mom

Mom, thanks for always believing in me and being my number one cheerleader. Your unconditional love and strength is amazing. Thank you also for being such a wonderful example on how to live life.

My Wife

Cara, You are an amazing wife, mother, and my best friend. Thanks for always believing in me and being my Rock!!

David McGarry

My Kids

Caitlynn and Adyson, you have your father wrapped around your finger and I wouldn't have it any other way. I hope the healthy lifestyle that your mother and I lead and the one we try to provide for your girls will be something you pass along to your kids. Keep being the amazing girls you are and know your Dad loves you!!

Contents

Foreword 1

Your First Challenge -
If You Choose to Accept 5

A Day That Shaped My Life 7

It's Your Choice 21

It's Not Rocket Science.. 27

Begin With the End in Mind 35

The Power of Changing One Thing 47

5 Habits to Get Fit 55

Fit Habit 1: Diet 59

Fit Habit 2: Exercise.. 69

Fit Habit 3: Sleep 77

Fit Habit 4: Accountability................................... 81

Fit Habit 5: Stay the Course 87

What's Next?... 91

My Fit Over 40 Inspiration 101

Take the Challenge.. 105

The Fit Over 40 Challenge Begins 109

6-Week Program 111

Message From David... 125

Foreword

IF YOU ARE READING this book then I am going to assume two things about you: 1) you are motivated to get healthier, and 2) you are over the age of forty.

David McGarry is one of the most passionate fitness professionals that I've had the privilege to know over the past twenty years. I met David in 1997 while working at the Cooper Fitness Center in Dallas, Texas, and the one thing I most admire about him is his passion to help others reach their optimum potential. This book is a great resource for anyone over the age of forty who wants to change their behavior in order to live a longer and healthier life. David's education and experience in the health, fitness and wellness arenas, along with his positive attitude and motivation to help others, is the perfect formula for success. The personal testimonies he shares in this book humanize the challenges we all face as we age and will inspire you to make the effort to change.

My name is Brad Wilkins, and I am the Senior Vice President of Operations at the Cooper Aerobics Center. It is interesting what happens to a person's perspective about life when they hit forty. For me, I started thinking more about my accomplishments, my goals, my dreams, my family, and my mortality. Reflecting on my own experiences and observations over the last four years since I turned forty, I've come to the conclusion it is the circumstances in life that seem to takes place during this time of one's life (like watching your parents age or pass on and your kids grow up to be more independent, or evaluating the job satisfaction you feel at the place of your employment and the goals you have or have not accomplished) that shapes us; because we are all creatures of habit driven by stimulus that bring us both joy and pain, going in cycles that are controlled by the emotions of everyday living.

Your health during your forties matters more than what is commonly understood. Research shows that the better shape you are in during this decade will tee you up for a longer, healthier life; because when a person dies, he or she dies not so much of the particular disease as of the behaviors of his or her entire life. So I encourage you to read this book, trust it, get up, and get started.

Your First Challenge - If You Choose to Accept

DID YOU FEEL LIKE you were Ethan Hunt (Tom Cruise) from Mission Impossible when you read that title? I love the part of the *Mission Impossible* movie series when the recorded message plays. Anyway, since you are an action taker, and decided to give this book a shot, I want to share with you a challenge you might be willing to accept. Most of us long to have a lean and strong core but have not had much success – partly because of the approach you have taken and also because of the misconception of what you think needs to be done to achieve it.

Don't worry though because I have created the "Six Days to a Stronger Core Challenge" to get you moving the in the right direction and finally get that leaner, stronger core you desire.

David McGarry

If you choose to accept the challenge, go to www.FitOver40Challenge.com/Core.

CHAPTER 1

A Day That Shaped My Life

On May 6, 2006, my life changed forever. I remember the day like it was yesterday. It was a warm Saturday morning with a Texas clear blue sky. I was up early that morning because it was moving day! We had sold our house six weeks earlier and were moving into an apartment while our new house was being built. After the birth of our first child, my wife and I decided it was a good time to move to a bigger home and start our life as a new family. Little did I know the stress of being a new dad and moving into a small apartment would have on me! But hey in Texas you either go big or go home, so we decided to go for it!

The movers arrived at my house, loaded everything up, and followed me to the apartment. My wife and baby daughter would meet me there later. Now I have to step back a second and also let you know why Saturdays were unique for me. My family lives in Florida and every Saturday morning since I moved to Texas my dad would call me. It didn't matter what was going on; he just wanted to catch up and see how things were going. He was so excited to hear how his new granddaughter was doing. This Saturday was no different, and sure enough, my phone started to ring as soon as I pulled into the apartment complex with the movers. I saw that it was my dad and thought about letting the call go to voicemail so I could have a minute to get the movers started, but something in me said *"You better take this call from your dad."* During our conversation, my dad sounded like he was sick, but he reassured me that everything was okay. We talked for a few minutes and reconfirmed his upcoming July visit to meet his new granddaughter.

That evening, I was relaxing after a long day of moving, and the phone rang. When my wife told me my Uncle Bob was on the line, I knew something was not right. I got on the phone and my uncle told me my dad had passed away from a major heart attack. He had been rushed him to the hospital, but they were unable to resuscitate him. He was only 67. I couldn't believe the news and then I just wept. The first thought that went through my mind was he never got to meet his new granddaughter. As the night went on, I had my ups and downs and then began to feel a little guilty. I started to blame myself for his death. Since I was a kid, I was always concerned about my dad's health, and I felt like it was my job to help him get fit and healthy. I remember always trying to get him to stop smoking, eat better, and work out. For years after he passed away, I thought surely I could have done something.

To his credit, he did try at times to make changes but he just had developed such poor habits over the years and changing them was not easy. I am not going to make excuses for my dad, but he did grow up in a time where there wasn't a lot of emphasis on health and fitness. People smoked, ate high-saturated foods, and didn't work out. So fitness and a healthy lifestyle never really became habits for him, and over the course of years, it took a big toll on him. He became extremely overweight, was a type 2 diabetic, struggled with back issues, and had a few minor strokes.

His passing, although shocking the day it happened, wasn't really a total surprise. I knew he did not have long to live because six months prior I visited him in Florida and went to the doctor with him. When the doctor told me that my father was too far gone on the other side, I knew that meant it was only a matter of time until something bad happened. Again, I always felt I could have done more to change him. It wasn't until years later I realized that ultimately I can't change somebody; they have to change themselves. However, I could still try to educate, motivate, and maybe make an impact in somebody's life that would change their bad habits and get them on the track to living a fit and healthy life. That Saturday in May changed my life forever and is a driving factor for writing this book.

Why I Wrote This Book

I know that I can only do so much, and everybody has to take responsibility for their actions, but what I have come to realize is that my God-given talent, or superpower, is to motivate others to become their best self and to give them the tools to change their habits and lifestyle. I may not have been able to change my father's habits, but over the years of training hundreds of clients, I have impacted many lives. However, I am always striving to do more and I want to share my superpower with those who are at the point where they want to change and will listen to a professional that has not only helped hundreds of people, but also practices what he preaches.

As we get older and move into our 40's, our bodies change and our metabolism begins to slow. Unfortunately, our bodies don't respond and recover the same way they did 10 or 20 years ago. Also, how you approach fitness and weight loss is much different in your 40's 50's than in your 20's and 30's.

I know I can't bring my father back, but I feel if I can change one person's life though this book and get them to take action and change their lifestyle and daily habits, then this book will have been a success.

The third reason I'm writing this book is for my kids. I know it is important to lead by example, and I want them to know being fit and healthy is important to me. When they see that, I hope it becomes important to them, and if they have kids, they lead by example and tell them about my coaching and the importance of being fit.

One goal I have for you while reading this book is that you figure out your "why" that you want to get fit and healthy once and for all.

Is This Book For You?

Let me be perfectly clear–if you are looking for the next big diet or next insane workout routine, then this book is not for you. Also, if you are already working out and looking for a more advanced routine or approach to losing weight, this will probably not be what you are looking for. However, you still might be able to take one or two things away from this book to incorporate into your daily life.

I know most people will be looking for some workouts to get them started and a step-by-step plan to incorporate into their daily routine. I will have that for you, but what you are also going to find in this book are strategies and habits that will help with long-term successful weight loss that I have used with my clients that have proven to work if implemented.

Just to reiterate, this is not some "Lose Weight Fast" approach so if you are looking for a "quick fix" or something that promises a new sexy body in six days, I suggest you look for another book. My whole purpose is to share my story and the approach I use in getting my clients to reach their goals.

The principles, strategies, and the challenge I will present at the end of the book can be put into place and used by anyone. The person I am speaking to, though, is the male or female who has spent the last few years in the their comfort zone and now feels frustrated with the way they look and feel about themselves and isn't really sure if they can be fit in their 40's.

I believe that you if you're age 40 or above, that does not mean you can't become fit or you can't get into the best shape of your life. However, the way you go about becoming fit may be different from when you were 20 or 30. Ultimately the decision is yours because you absolutely can become fit again, and you can live a very healthy life. For those of you who have tried everything else and failed, I am going to ask you to go through this book and read some of the proven strategies I have used with my clients over the years of coaching. Don't quit on yourself. You are probably closer to success than you realize!

Why You Should Listen To Me

I know that you could not care less about how many certifications I have, how many people

I've trained, or how many years I've been coaching. What you really want to know is whether or not I can provide you the solutions you're looking for. I want to take just a moment and tell you a little bit about who I am and why I believe what I have to say to you in this book will be the answers to your questions and frustration for not seeing long term results.

Who am I? My name is David McGarry. I am a trainer and coach who has been helping transform others not only on the outside, but also on the inside, for just over two decades. I have worked with all types of clients who have different goals and reasons for using my services. I am not a celebrity coach and I haven't trained any actors or actresses. I haven't created a new hyped-up diet plan where you can lose 20 lbs. in 10 days by doing such and such. I am an ordinary coach that over the past 20+ years has helped my clients implement simple daily habits and lifestyle changes transforming their lives for the long haul.

My clients who have seen the best results have not become obsessive gym rats, but rather more disciplined individuals who follow daily habits and, more importantly, change their lifestyle and mental attitude towards being fit and healthy. Looking back and studying the clients who achieved the biggest results, I discovered their results were not achieved with some hyped up diet plan or crazy workout plan like "4 minutes to flat, sexy, strong, rock solid, six pack abs," but were achieved with shifts into being more disciplined by following healthy habits, lifestyle changes and changing mindsets. Not only did I study the results of my previous clients to come up with my proven strategies for success, but I myself am also living proof that simple changes in your life can really work.

When I first thought about writing this book, I knew I could share my knowledge as a fitness professional, but I also felt it was important for me to be transparent and upfront about my fitness journey. I face the same struggles as you. As hard as I try to lead by example, I am also human. I give in to temptations. I lack discipline at times. I sometimes lack the motivation to do the things I need to do to see change.

When I was close to turning 40, I found myself in the worst shape of my life and I was comfortable with the status quo. You may be wondering why you should listen to someone who has struggled and continues to struggle with the same problems you are facing. Well, I understand that thought and, to be honest, it is not something that I am proud of, but I don't want to hide from it either. Part of planning for success is admitting past shortcomings, and when you do, then you can finally move forward.

So, what exactly do I believe led to this? In my mid 30's I was fired from my job and decided to start my own business. On top of that, my wife and I had two young toddlers that kept us busy, and I did not make my own fitness a major priority. My clothes no longer fit, and I just didn't have the same energy and confidence I had ten years earlier. Then a friend of mine asked me to come check out a new workout facility where she was working. It was an amazing workout and class. I absolutely loved it because it put everything together in terms of workout, accountability, the group atmosphere, and the science of exercise.

I've been in the fitness industry for a long time and I have seen fitness fads come and go, but this class was set up to get you into the proper heart rate zones that allow you to burn calories hours after the workout is complete which is referred to as EPOC (Excess Post-exercise Oxygen Consumption), or informally called "The Afterburn."

After taking this class, I realized how much I missed that euphoria and high I got from having an amazing workout. We didn't do anything revolutionary, but I realized that I was not pushing myself and I was just going through the motions and checking my workout off my to-do list. After that workout, I started to reflect and wondered what am I really doing and am I living the life of a healthy and fit individual? I figured I had a choice. I could either start practicing what I preach and believe, or suffer the consequences down the road and maybe end up with the same fate as my father.

That started a chain reaction, and I began to think about how I wanted to live out the rest of my life and what I wanted my life to be like 20, 30 or, if I am lucky, 40 years from now. I knew I needed to change my fitness habits for my kids. I want to watch them grow old and be there for them. If my kids have their own kids, I want to be able to spend an entire day at Disney with them, like my mother did with her grandkids at the age of 73. If I had not changed my habits and fitness, I might have struggled to keep up with my kids and stay at the park for as long as we did. I know for a fact that if I were not in good shape in my 70's, there would be no way I could do what my mom did that day.

I finally made the decision that my health and well being was much more than "*I want to look good and fit back in my clothes.*" Don't get me wrong... that can be a goal, but you need to have a greater reason and purpose behind being fit and healthy for it to become a lasting change.

I've made my reasons clear, but if your reasons unclear and you just aren't sure what your "why" is, don't worry, I'm going to help you find it a little later in the book. Also, I hope by telling you my story and struggles, you understand that I am exactly like you in one way. I have to continuously work and make it a priority to stay fit and to stay in shape. I am proud to tell you that after being in the worst shape of my life a few years ago, I am now probably in the best shape of my life. How did I do it? I did exactly what I preach to my clients and continuously go back to my "why" when I want to quit or get off track!

CHAPTER 2

It's Your Choice

You Can Make the Choice

Each day, you make many choices—likely more than you realize. You can choose to make today a great day, or you can choose to look at today through a cloud, and not have a good day. You choose what clothes to wear and the route you take to work. You may even choose how you go about getting your work done. Everything you do is a choice.

Your health is a choice too. How do you want to look and feel? Will you continue to do nothing, feel miserable, have little energy and complain that your clothes do not fit correctly? It is your choice whether you work out or not. So, how you look and feel is up to you.

Have you ever wished that you could change something in your life right this moment? I believe that changes can happen in a moment—in the blink of an eye, in fact.

While some people believe that change is something that takes weeks, months or years to achieve and that you must try and fail many times before success occurs, that isn't always the case. When you are truly committed to the choice, the change occurs instantly, even if it takes some time for the results to show themselves fully.

Do you know many people who have struggled with their weight, want to get in shape but can't seem to make the change?

Are their things in your life you want to change—such as weight you want to lose, high blood pressure you want to lower, or a pair of pants you would like to be able to wear? What prevents you from making these positive changes?

Self-help guru Tony Robbins once said, "It's the getting ready to change that takes time. In the end, there's a single instant when the change occurs." In the documentary based on his famed "Date with Destiny" seminar, Tony speaks three beliefs that are necessary to make an instant and lasting change, if you want to reach success. I've summarized this information below. This can be a strategy to help you make these important changes in your life.

Believe That Something Must Change

There is a difference between "wanting to get in shape" and knowing that you must lose weight. Have you reached the end of your rope? To make a lasting change, you should be aware that the time for change has arrived.

Believe That You Must Be the One to Change It

While others may help, you are going to be the one that makes it happen. You have to be ready to make this a personal mission and realize that no one will do it for you.

Believe That You Can Change It

You have to let past failures go. When you put your mind to it, you have to know that you can lose weight or make any other positive choice in your life. Knowing yourself goes a long way towards helping you succeed.

Why do many people fail when they aim to make a change like this? They depend on willpower to do it. While this may work for a little while, the time will come when they revert to what is comfortable. That is why success slips away, at least for the long haul.

Beat This by Changing What Is Comfortable

Most people are motivated by two things—avoiding pain and gaining pleasure. If you want to change your behavior, you need to associate pain with your non-desired behavior and pleasure with your desired behavior.

To lose weight, you need to stop eating comfort food (especially late at night). You also want to exercise regularly. This is what the basics of weight loss come down to—eating less and working out more. Previously, you found comfort food pleasurable and exercise painful so you avoided the things that were good for you.

It is time to retrain your brain so that it feels good about exercising and bad about late night binges and fatty comfort foods. Think about all those negative things about being overweight and connect those thoughts to a late night snack. You do not want to feel good when you sit down to an unhealthy late night snack do you?

On the other hand, you want to be able to think about how wonderful it would be to be in shape and connect those thoughts to exercise. This is when you want to feel your best—when you are working out and improving yourself. Later in this book, I will expand on the aforementioned beliefs and provide strategies that you can use after you have begun your quest for health. After all, I feel like you are ready to change, or you wouldn't be reading this book.

CHAPTER 3

It's Not Rocket Science

LET'S FACE IT, we all know that in order to lose weight we need to exercise and eat right. Knowing how to lose weight isn't rocket science, however, even though we know what we need to do to lose weight, our society as a whole has become more obese. Before I had the idea to write this book, I started to reflect back over the years of coaching clients and thought about why some had major transformations and lost weight but others did not. What I realized was the success they achieved in regards to their weight loss was due to a few simple habits and lifestyle choices that they implemented into their daily lives. It had nothing to do with some crazy diet I came up with or some crazy workout plan.

It really came down to figuring out their "why," creating S.M.A.R.T. goals, implementing healthy habits, and overall lifestyle change. Some people want a quick fix, but I am not here to come up with the latest fad. I am here to be upfront and honest about what it takes to transform your body and your life so as you age you continue to be fit and live a functional life! For those of you who are willing to take the path least traveled, or the slow but steady path,

I am going to share those simple strategies with you. I honestly believe if you follow these strategies, you're going to see results and, if you stick with it, you will transform yourself for the rest of your life.

The first step starts with you believing that something has to change. Regardless of how many times you have tried to lose weight or get fit, you have to begin to believe it is possible and that this time it is going to happen. The body follows what the mind believes is possible and until you start believing that you can and will lose weight, you will struggle.

Once you believe and know that you must change, you have to dig deep and define your why. Why do you want to lose weight? It can't be because you want your clothes to fit better. That is too superficial and doesn't acknowledge the real issues behind your need to lose weight. You need to probe a little further and ask why do you want to get into the clothes that no longer fit you? Are you going to feel more attractive? Do you think your spouse will look at you the way they did when you first got married? Do you want to have more energy so you are able to play with your kids longer?

You've got to really dig deep and find the real reason for wanting to make change! I have found that my clients who had a strong "why" made it through the challenging times. When they felt like quitting, their "why" brought them back into focus and they kept going!

So how do you come up with your "why?" In order to find your "why," you really have to get down to where the pain is. You may ask what pain I am referring to. Well, let's say that the reason you want to lose weight is to look good. It can't be that you just want to look good. It has to be something bigger. There is a reason you want to look better and that is where the pain is. Maybe looking better is going to make you feel sexy again and attractive to your spouse. The pain is that you no longer feel good about yourself physically and losing the extra 10-15 lbs. will give you confidence and make you feel attractive. The goal of losing weight to look good is fine, but you have to establish the bigger reason and that becomes your "why!' Let's look at some specific examples of clients I have worked with.

Client #1

Years after we stopped training together, a good friend and former client told me that establishing his "why" led to his transformation. This is was an "Aha" moment for me and is the reason I am putting so much emphasis on knowing your why. Once you have it, it can lead to your success!

When I first started working with him, he had never had an organized work out before in his life in terms of weight training or a weight loss program. I always begin with any client by having an initial consultation. I asked, "Why do you want to work out now? You haven't done it before, so why now?" After talking for several minutes he realized he wanted to do it for his kids! He was getting older he didn't have the energy and stamina he once had when he was younger. He wanted to be physically able to be active with his kids. He wanted to be to the point where if his kids wanted to go out and run around, he would be able to do it.

As simple as that sounds, it was so much bigger than "*Hey, I just wanted to lose weight and look good and feel good.*" Again, I'm not saying there's anything wrong with that, but his "why" was bigger than him. It had everything to do with his kids, which was also similar to my why. I decided to make my health and fitness a huge priority because of my family and my desire to be active with my kids as they continue to grow up. Sometimes when we make our reasons for doing something to be more than just about ourselves, we become more motivated to actually make it happen and to stay the course!

Client #2

This person wasn't new to working out, but someone who worked out a few times a week in the gym. She always wanted to take her fitness to another level, but didn't know how to get there. I noticed when we first met that she never had a strong drive or motivation to do the things it took to get there.

During our initial consultation, I asked her several questions about her prior exercise history, injuries, and reasons for her goals, which eventually led us to coming up with her "why." She ultimately decided that she wanted to do this because she wanted to feel accomplished and do something that she had never done before. She had accomplished a lot of great things in her professional career, but had sacrificed her fitness while focusing on all of her professional accomplishes. Establishing her "why" motivated her to ultimately start running triathlons. Once she reached that goal she started doing half marathons, and eventually the bigger goal of marathons! She gives me credit for it, but actually it just came down to figure out her pain point and ultimately her "why!"

Now it is time for a little homework. I want you to spend some time thinking about your "why" and what is the real pain behind your desire to get fit and healthy. Once you have that in your mind, write it down and put it somewhere that you will see daily. It needs to get etched into your mind every day. When you figure that out, it's going to change your mindset and your purpose to "*Hey, this isn't just about me, it's about something else.*" This is the first step in your successful fitness journey.

CHAPTER 4

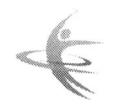

Begin With the End in Mind

When we look at creating different mindsets and shifts in the way we think, one of the things we have to do is get some clarity so we have the vision of what it is we want. We've already determined the "why" and know why you're going to do it, but really get clear on what is it that you want out of your life.

So what am I talking about here? Well, I was first exposed to this mindset shift when I graduated college. I read the book *The Seven Habits of Highly Successful People* by Stephen Covey. I started to follow one of his—to live a great life, you have to know what exactly you want from life and do that. You need to begin with the end in mind. When I first read that, I had an "Aha" moment. I began to ask myself, "What do I want from my life? If it ends tomorrow, would my obituary encompass all my accomplishments?" When I answered that question, I had a complete turnaround in my life. I decided that I needed to stop just being comfortable and needed to start challenging myself. I also decided that when I am 85 or 90, assuming I live that long, I want to be active. I want to be able to walk on my own, drive, and still live a very good quality life. Without your health, you will be severely limited to what you can do and can't do as you get older. The problem with the world today is we are living longer, but our quality of life is declining due to self-causing diseases and disabilities.

Once you determine what you want your life to be like when you are in your so-called "Golden Years," I want you to take the next step. Start to visualize yourself where you want to be at the end of your life, or as Stephen Covey writes in his book *The Seven Habits of Highly Successful People* to begin with the end in mind. You have to know what you want out of life. Do you want to travel when you retire? Do you want to be able to play with your grandkids or take them on trips? Once you have an idea of what you what your life to be like when you older, then you have to come back to reality and ask yourself, how are you going to get there? Is the lifestyle you are living and the healthy habits you are practicing going to get you there. If not, then you need to make a change and you can start by changing the way you think and what you believe.

Mind Shift and Mantras

The reason I want you to find your "why" and figure out the kind of health you want for your life is that I believe mindset is responsible for 95% of the success we achieve. You need to be able to control the thoughts and beliefs you have going on inside your head if you want to see results. There are plenty of temptations and distractions to take you off course from being fit, but if you are constantly keeping your mind focused on the right messages and capabilities, then you will win the race! You may find yourself struggling with negative thoughts from time to time. Here are some simple strategies for dealing with unwanted thoughts and those feelings of failure.

First, whenever you experience a disempowering thought, gently push it away (without judgment) and replace it with one or more of the following mantras that are listed below. Also, reflect on your mantras for at least 15-30 seconds and feel the emotional sensations that come along with the words. Finally, only choose mantras that resonate with your mission. You must believe them to be true or else your emotions will repel your subconscious mind from creating the desired result.

Then, repeat your favorite mantras for at least five minutes prior to going to sleep and five minutes after waking (**before** checking your phone or doing anything else). This is when your brain waves are still in their most subconscious state. Take advantage of this opportunity to get specific about what you desire.

- I am beautiful/handsome.
- I am a healthy and energetic person.
- I accept me, each and every cell of who I am.
- I am safe. I release all beliefs that are blocking me from (insert your goal).
- I allow myself to be fit.
- Reaching my ideal weight is easy and fun.
- I am open to losing weight and seeing myself in a new healthy body. I deserve it.
- I am excited to nourish my body with healthy food.
- My body reflects what an extraordinary and unique person I am.

I know it may seem strange and you may want to dismiss it, but repeating those mantras and shifting your thoughts to positive thoughts and feelings really can make a huge difference in your success. I am not a psychologist, but one thing that has always fascinated me is the power of the subconscious mind. The subconscious mind cannot reason like the conscious mind can and not only have I read about amazing stories of people overcoming disease and other ailments, I have seen it first hand with myself and clients. Even just on a superficial level when I wake up and start my day with positive daily mantras, I have a totally different feeling and energy about the day. So do me a favor and quit looking at Facebook and your social media when you first wake up and start saying your daily mantras and shift your mind to positive thoughts to start your day and week! Try it for 30 days and tell me you didn't see any results!

Goals

Shifting your mindset and feeding yourself with positive thoughts is a good first step. However, you need to set some clear goals. If you don't know what you want, then how are you going to set a plan to get there? One of the coaches I work with says, "*A day without a goal is a day wasted!*" I thought that was pretty powerful because unfortunately there are a lot of people who just wake up and let the day happen to them. Before you know it, a decade or two goes by and you never accomplish what you wanted.

If you are like most people, you set short or long-term goals on New Year's, but after a few short weeks of not being consistent and seeing results, you drop off. In years past, I used to be just like everyone else. Typically starting in late November and December I would spend several hours reviewing my previous goals from the past year and then set goals for the upcoming year. It went something like this, maybe you can relate, "*I want to lose five to ten pounds by the end of the year, so by December 31st, I want to be such and such weight.*" Does that sound familiar to your approach? Don't worry, I did the same thing and I am not saying you can't get results by doing that approach, but I want to introduce you to an approach I started doing about a year ago.

I was introduced to Brian Moran's book titled *The 12 Week Year*. In the book, Moran details how every 12 weeks you establish your goals for a 12-week period and after 12 weeks, you review your goals. If you didn't reach your goal, you either revise it for the next 12 weeks or maybe scratch it all together. Moran points out in his book that the longer time frame associated with a goal, the less likely you are to get after it and the more likely you are to procrastinate until the deadline gets closer. For instance, if you are in sales you probably know that the 4th quarter of the year is usually crunch time and most companies really make a push to meet their goals then. The same is true for those of us setting fitness and weight loss goals. If we set a goal to lose ten pounds by the end of the year, or even six months (bathing suit season if you start on Jan 1), the tendency is to procrastinate. If you don't get right after it, you know you still have more time and put it off until later.

By setting more manageable, frequent goals, I found more success. Instead of giving myself an entire year to lose ten pounds and procrastinating, I became more disciplined and focused on the task I had ahead of me. There's nothing wrong with having a long-term goal or vision, especially if you have a lot of weight to lose, but you want to break it down and start setting 12-week goals for yourself.

Another benefit to following the "12-week year" plan is if after a few weeks, you blow it and go back to the same bad habits, you will forget about your goals until the end of the year. However, breaking your goals down to 12 weeks gives you a fresh start every 12 weeks regardless of your level of success. No matter how disciplined you are and how committed you are to reaching your goals, you are going to blow it at some point. You are human and even the people you think are the most seriously disciplined people have bad days and even bad weeks. Life sometimes just gets in the way. But, if you use a 12-week approach, you get to start over, reassess and go for it again.

Think about baseball players. No player will bat 1,000 every day. A really good hitter is lucky to bat .300. That means he is getting a hit three out of every ten at bats. The same is true with you. You are not going to win every day and reach every goal. If you begin to create goals that center around a 12-week time frame and fall short, all you have to do is set another 12-week goal instead of feeling defeated and quitting all together. So, change your mindset and process by having a "New Year" every 12 weeks!

Now that we have a new fresh mindset on goal setting, I want to walk you through the process of setting up a truly successful goal. You have probably set goals for yourself in the past and you're thinking, "*Well how hard can it be?*" The biggest mistakes I see people make when they set goals for themselves is that they don't set S.M.A.R.T. (Specific, Measurable, Attainable, Realistic, and Timely) goals. What is so different and special about this type of goal setting? Well, a lot of times when I meet with a new client they give me really vague and weak goals. Let me walk you through a sample conversation with a typical client.

"Dave, I really want to lose weight."
"Okay, great. How much weight?
"Oh, at least 10-15 pounds."
"Okay, and in what time frame?"

"I want to do it next week."

"Well, that's not really realistic."

"Can it be done in six weeks?"

"Yes, that is more realistic!"

In that scenario, you can see how I get the client to dig a little deeper and set a more realistic goal with a time frame. Now, let's take a look at what I would suggest if weight loss is your goal. Let's say you want to lose 15 pounds. Now we have the measurable part down and it is somewhat specific. Let's continue through the process to see if it is reasonable and timely. This is where people get tripped up and set themselves up for failure. We live in an "I want it today society" and people don't set realistic expectations. If I set a goal for myself to lose 15 pounds, I would say one lb. per week would be healthy, which would put me at about 15 weeks. However, it is possible to lose one to two lbs. per week and still be healthy, so we could set up a more aggressive goal. If you were to set a 12-week goal, you would have to lose 1.25 lbs. per week. That is very realistic and obtainable while at the same time safe.

Here is what the goal would look like if I were to start on January 1st and plan for a 12-week period.

I, David McGarry, will lose 15 pounds and weigh 190 lbs. on March 31st.

One last point to make here is you need to have deadlines. Setting a goal for 12 weeks puts a deadline on you to get it done. The sample goal I presented above has all of the elements of being specific, measurable, attainable, realistic and timely. So now it is your turn. Set up your S.M.A.R.T. goal and share it with me at dave@davemcgarry.com or in the Health and Fitness accountability group, which you can join for FREE at

Facebook.com/Groups/AllAboutHealthAndFitness

CHAPTER 5

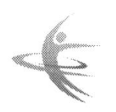

The Power of Changing One Thing

As we continue down this journey, I hope you are beginning to see that I am laying out the plan for you to set yourself up for success on being fit over 40. Planning is great, but if we fail to take action and implement what we learn then we won't see the results. I am going to start laying out the strategies and habits that you need to start taking that eventually will become your new lifestyle. If you implement these simple daily habits, you will start to see results and will have the success you are looking for.

The first action I want you to take is to pick one thing and get rid of it. This is what I call the power of changing one thing! What do I mean by the power of changing one thing? Well, sometimes we think that in order to make a change in our habits or lifestyle it needs to be drastic, but the tendency is to fall right back into the same old bad habits and routine. So instead of getting too crazy all at once, I want you to think of one thing that you are currently consuming that you know either contains too much sugar, like a 12 oz. Coke, or something that is high in empty calories.

Fit Over 40 Challenge

The secret to losing weight is simple. Make small changes and losing weight starts to compound over time. The Power of just "One Thing" can make a huge difference. Let's look at an example:

Let's say you go to Starbucks every morning and buy a Grande Latte. Now, depending upon how you have it prepared, the calorie content will vary. See below:

- Starbucks Cafe Latte prepared with nonfat milk–160 calories
- Starbucks Cafe Latte prepared with soy–210 calories
- Starbucks Cafe Latte prepared with whole milk–60 calories

*Based on approximate calorie content (Grande size) provided by Starbucks.com

Now we will make a small change and do the math. Cut out the Café Latte that is prepared with whole milk from our daily intake. This cuts a total of 260 calories each day.

260 x 7 = 1,820 calories per week

Multiply 1,820 calories per week by 26 weeks (six months) = 47,320 calories

Now divide that by 3500 calories, which is one pound of fat and you could potentially lose 13.5 lbs. by making the choice to cut out that daily drink.

Also, since I am advocating that you break down your goals into 12-week periods, let's look at the impact you can make it that time period.

260 x 7 = 1,820 calories per week

Multiply, 1,820 per week by 12 weeks = 21,840 calories. If you divide that number by 3,500 calories, one pound of fat, you could lose almost 6.5 pounds in a 12-week period.

I hope you are beginning to see the power of making one small change and what a difference it can make.

80/20 Principle

I want to take what I just shared with you and expand upon it and share another strategy that can help you get results. Have you ever heard about the 80/20 principle? Some of you might be familiar with this as it's widely used in a business sense. It's also known as the Pareto Principle and it's commonly talked about in the sales world. Essentially, the 80/20 principle means that 20% of your efforts is going to result in 80% of your results.

So, how does this apply to fitness? Well, I know everyone is pressed for time and most people live very busy lives, so if you want to maximize your time and efforts you need to focus in on the small things, that 20%, that will have the biggest impact on your lifestyle and in your daily routines, ultimately giving you 80% of the results. A lot of times we think we need to work out for two to three hours a week to get us the results we want. Your daily workout is 4% of your day so what else are you going to do the other 96% that can make a huge impact on your efforts? That is where your daily habits and lifestyle choices come into play. If you were to examine your daily lifestyle and habits, what are you doing that's sabotaging the results you want?

Here's a quick example of a small change that can make an 80/20 impact. When I was younger, I would drink eight to ten ounces of orange juice every morning. As a kid, I would drink so much orange juice that I'd break out in hives! As a young adult, I knew that drinking that much orange juice with all the sugar it contained was one reason I was not losing weight, but was gaining weight. Even though I loved my orange juice, I knew I had to tweak my diet and I cut it out from my morning routine. I went cold turkey one day and made the decision it would no longer be a daily ritual! It wasn't easy, but the way I looked at it was that I was cutting out 150 calories in my diet every day! I know it's not a lot, but I now have a caloric deficit of 150 calories, and so after a certain period of time, I knew I would start to lose weight. It doesn't seem like a lot, but if we are following the 12-week goal setting technique, it is about 21,840 calories. To lose weight you need to have a caloric deficit of 3500, so divide that and in a six month time frame that would be over 7.2 lbs. if all you do is reduce your daily caloric deficit by 150 calories a day. That is the power behind making one small change to your diet or daily lifestyle.

Your 20% change can be as simple as cutting out as much daily sugar intake as possible. Follow me on this line of thinking. What if your daily sugar intake is high and you reduce the amount of sugar you take in a day? If you're a Coke drinker and you stop drinking Cokes, that could be at least a 200 to 300 daily caloric reduction just from sugar. Do you know what kind of impact that is going to have on your weight loss and lifestyle? It shouldn't be too difficult to do. Well, maybe initially it is, but it wasn't like you had to put in a crazy amount of effort. That 20% effort that you put in to reduce sugar from your daily diet can turn out to be responsible for 80% of your results. That is the 80/20 principle at work and I hope you see the power it can have on you reaching your fitness and weight loss goals!

5 Habits to Get Fit

IF YOU WANT TO get fit and stay fit, it all comes down to habits. The number one question I get asked is, "*How can I quickly and easily get fit?*" If you have read this far into the book, you should know by now that there is no quick and easy way, If you want to change your lifestyle and be in this journey for the long run, focus on five habits that highly successful and fit people do every day that help them reach their health and fitness goals.

1. Diet

I really hate to sound stale or not have anything revolutionary to add here, but nutrition is probably 95% of the ball game. It's not about calorie counting or a particular diet, it's about eating the proper foods and nutrients.

2. Exercise

Unfortunately we live in a time period where technology is amazing, but it is also leading to the current obesity problem we are experiencing. We are becoming more sedentary and less movement-oriented as a whole. I would argue that most people don't even realize how little movement they do throughout the day and then when they do exercise, it is not enough to get them into the proper zones to burn fat and speed up their metabolism.

3. Sleep

A lot of people neglect this one, but sleep is extremely important when it comes to overall health. It has been shown to actually affect weight gain and weight loss. Plus, it is important for general health and your overall energy levels.

4. Accountability

This one is one of those steps that people tend to neglect or not take seriously. I am not sure why, but my guess is they're a little bit embarrassed and they don't want people to know their shortcomings. Another reason is I think people don't realize the power behind having accountability and how it will help with their overall success. If you have ever listened to people who achieve success, they will usually mention that accountability played a role.

5. Stay the Course

My fitness journey has been like a roller coaster. If you're reading this, your journey probably has been as well. What I tend to see with clients or others wanting to lose weight and be fit is that if they have a bad couple of days or maybe a couple of weeks in terms of eating bad and not working out, it throws them off completely and they decide to stop and not get right back after it.

It is important to understand that being fit and healthy is a marathon and not a sprint. You are not going to win everyday and you might not win every week or month. However, it is important to stay the course because in the long run you will put together days that you win and those days add up and have an exponential effect on your overall health and well being! Giving up should never be an option. If you do fall off, get back up and start again as it will make a difference when everything is said and done.

CHAPTER 6

Fit Habit 1: Diet

YOU MAY ALREADY KNOW why it is important to focus on your diet. Unhealthy eating habits have contributed to the obesity epidemic in the United States, and it's said that 1/3 of U.S. adults are obese and approximately 17% (12.5 million) children and adolescents aged 2 to 19 are obese. That's pretty staggering and depressing if you ask me. Even for people of healthy weight, a poor diet is associated with major health risks and can cause illness and even death.

Typically when I first meet with a new client, I tell them that nutrition is about 90% of the equation when it comes to losing weight. Most of the time, the client says, "I know." If that's the case, then shouldn't it be pretty clear what needs to be done and what you should eat and not eat? Unfortunately, the answer is no and there are several reasons for this. One reason is there is a lot of misinformation out there. Another reason is the hyped up diets and marketing that goes on in the diet and fitness industry. Finally, the last reason is due to the type of foods we consume. A lot of the foods people eat daily are processed, contain high amounts of sugar, and are carbohydrate-based. When you eat foods like these, the pancreas releases insulin. Insulin is what controls the amount of glucose (sugar) levels that transfer from your blood into your cells. Basically, excess glucose in your cells turns into fat cells. So when we overeat (especially certain types of carbs like starchy breads, pasta and other refined carbohydrates like white rice), excess glucose enters our cells and turns into fat cells for your body to use later.

Another important point to make here is as we age, the way we metabolize and process our food changes. You may be saying, *"But in my twenties and thirties it didn't matter what I ate."* That may be true, but your body changes as you get older so it is more important now than ever to limit the amount of refined carbohydrates and processed foods.

So, if you want to maintain or even lose weight, you have to control your insulin levels. To do that, you need to control the amount of food (i.e., calories) you eat and avoid certain types of carbs like pasta, potatoes, and other refined "fast carbs" like white rice. I am not saying eliminate them all together because me being Italian, I love pasta, but make sure you are measuring and eating the right serving size.

That's the somewhat technical explanation of why we get fat and simple way to lose weight.

The next question you may be asking is how much food should you eat? You might recall earlier I said it's not about calorie counting for the people that I've seen who have lost weight and kept it off. You need to understand your metabolic rate. Your metabolic rate is important because in working with clients whose goals have been to lose weight, they often approach it all wrong. The first thing they do is go on a starvation diet. This reduces their calories to the point where they aren't eating enough to maintain the lean muscle tissue they currently have.

Essentially, if you stop feeding your body and put it into starvation mode, you are going to shut the body down from using its energy sources (think fat). It's going to go directly to the easiest source of energy, which is your muscle tissue. I know it seems counterintuitive, but starving yourself is only going to work to a point and then your body shuts down from using fat as an energy source and uses your muscles that you are attempting to build.

Having a basic understanding of your ideal caloric intake is critical if your goal is weight loss, and of course, the American Diet Association recommends different amounts for males and females. Everybody is different and you also need to consider how much activity you're taking in. For example, at my current weight and activity level, my daily caloric intake should be around 2470. People vary depending on their current weight, metabolism, and activity. So you might be anywhere from 1800 - 2100 calories a day in order to properly fuel your body. If you're really active and you have a lot of lean muscle, you might take in 3000+ calories a day. The point I am trying to make is that you need to know how many calories you need to take in to help fuel your body and allow it to burn fat, which ultimately gets the weight loss you are looking for. If you aren't sure what your daily caloric intake should be, you can use the calculator on my website at

www.FitOver40Challenge.com/BookResources.

Once you know your Resting Metabolic Rate, the next thing to focus on is what you should be eating. Again, this is not a diet book, but my goal here is for you to understand that if you are taking in sensible nutrients, eating clean from natural food sources, and getting in the proper amount of calories, you will see results. Also, make sure you are taking in enough protein, carbohydrates, fats, and yes I'm talking about good fats. I know most "diets" will have you eliminate one particular group or be heavily concentrated on one to lose weight, but if you stick to eating meals with protein, carbs and essential fats, you will not go wrong. For myself, I follow a 45% carb, 35% protein, and 20% fats withe my daily intake of calories. There are many other recommendations and I believe it is not a one-size-fits-all approach with an individual's diet. You need to figure out what works best for you. To find out, you can do the trial and error method or get an RMR test done to find out if your body burns more carbs or fats at rest. Many places provide this service, so you can Google it or look to see if your area has a company called *Dexafit* nearby. The way you choose to get your numbers doesn't matter, but use one method to get them.

Once you have this information, it will help you understand what fuel source your body uses at rest. For instance, I burn a mixture of carbohydrates and fats. Ideally, I want to burn fat so I know that several workouts during the week I need to spend a greater amount of my workout in my aerobic or cardio zone. I also know how many calories I burn at rest, which allows me to know how many calories I should be consuming on a daily basis after I account for basic activity and lifestyle.

By using this information, I can track my caloric intake and know how many calories I need to maintain weight or lose weight. Without this information, I would just be guessing. Don't be lazy and make the mistake of just guessing if you want to see results.

Additionally, if you're frequently eating out at fast food restaurants, there's no way you're going to eat well. Often, the fast food salads have more calories and a higher fat content than a hamburger does. Be really strict in terms of where you're going out to eat, what is in your house, in your food, and your pantry, and your refrigerator.

Finally, when we talk about diet, we need to talk about how to track your diet. This is not about calorie counting or a specific diet, but initially you need to track what you're eating. Knowledge is power and after writing down and journaling your food intake for a week, you can get a great assessment if you are eating enough calories and how long are you going without eating in between meals.

If you are using an app, you might be able to calculate how much protein, sugar, and fat you are ingesting each day. This is an important exercise to do because it can give you insight into what you need to do change your daily diet and also get a snapshot of your reality as opposed to what you thought. So, to be blunt you need to understand what you're eating if you want to change.

There are several ways you can go about tracking your daily food intake. You can do the "old school" method and use a writing journal that you carry with you. A more high-tech way to do it would be to download an app to your smart phone. I have done it both ways but since my phone is always with me, I use an app. I personally like My Fitness Pal which allows you to track your meals, exercise and water intake. Another app I have used is FatSecret. The benefit to using an app is they have made it really simple to get all the information you need by scanning the barcode of the food item you are ingesting, or by searching in their database. I have heard that most people who track their food only will do this for less than a week and then stop. That is ok as our ultimate goal is to find out what you're putting in your body on a daily basis, what times of day you're eating, and how many total calories consumed. So, even if this is just for a week then that is ok. Just make sure you get that insight and knowledge because I will bet it will be an eye-opening experience for you.

CHAPTER 7

Fit Habit 2: Exercise

OUR SOCIETY HAS BECOME more and more sedentary. Technology has allowed us to do things that make us more inactive. In the past, many of things that we had to do required a lot more movement and energy, but now we've become more sedentary. Because of that, we're at risk for weight gain, which can lead to other issues like heart disease and Type 2 Diabetes. I recently read a statistic that less than 5% of the U.S. population had Type 2 Diabetes in 1990, but as of this writing (2016) it is now over 7%, which is a 40% increase! Wow! Unfortunately, most of this is due to the technological advances that we've had.

Today more people have jobs that require them to sit at a desk for hours at a time. We now have remote control TVs and smartphones that can turn appliances on and off making for a more sedentary lifestyle. Our bodies were actually meant to move and built to do "work." Since we have become less active, it is even more important to move and get exercise than ever before. Exercising is important, obviously for many reasons, but besides it helping you prevent a sedentary lifestyle, it also gives you energy. I run across this all the time with my clients. They often express to me that they are tired before a training session, but afterwards they tell me they feel better and more energetic and are glad they worked out.

You may be wondering how much exercise you need to be doing – and I think this is where people feel like, *Oh my gosh, I'm going to have to work out six days a week and I'm going to have to be at the gym for over an hour, well I just don't have the time for that.* First, I will say that you need to make changes to your daily routine. For example, instead of circling around the parking lot looking for the closest spot to the door, park your car farther away. Do the same at the office. Instead of taking the elevator, take the stairs. These small changes may seem insignificant, but in the long run can pay out big dividends. Once, you have made those small changes to your lifestyle, what really you need to focus in on is squeezing in moderate to high intensity exercise, three to four times a week. It doesn't have to be for an hour every time you work out. It could be for 30 minutes. Recent studies have shown you can get results with 30 minutes of high intensity interval training. Again, if you can get an hour in, that's going to be a little bit more beneficial for you.

I would combine the high-intensity interval training with resistance training, because you need to have resistance training, too. The reason why that's important is because as we get older, we lose lean muscle mass at a faster rate. For females, bone density is extremely important, so you want to do resistance training to not only help with bone density, but also to get lean and speed up your metabolism. Please, if you have the notion in your head that lifting weights is going to make you huge, get rid of that thought. Unless you are taking high dosages of testosterone, you will not build up large muscles. I know the first thing you think of when it comes to losing weight is to do cardio, but I promise lifting weights can be the difference maker when it comes to losing weight. At the end of this book, I will present you with a six-week challenge with some beginning exercises and resistance training to get your started.

I talked briefly about resistance training and mentioned HIIT training, but what is HIIT training? HIIT training is an acronym for High

Intensity Interval Training. Research shows that if you want to lose weight and speed up your metabolism, then it is important to get your heart rate to be in the higher zones. I am referring to the different cardiovascular zones obtained through exercise. You may have heard the terms "fat burning" zone, "aerobic zone" and "anaerobic zone." The mistake most people make is they do not get their heart rate in these different zones and although they are getting into their so called "aerobic zone," they are not getting their heart rate into the upper zones and therefore missing out on E.P.O.C. That is a big fancy word for creating the "afterburn" effect, which essentially allows you to burn calories 12-36 hours after the workout. One thing you need to take into consideration is you should always recover, hence the reason they say interval training. You do not want to always stay in the upper zones without bringing the heart rate back down because if you stay too long in higher heart rate zones, it can end up being counterproductive.

So, how do you figure out your zones so you can track it? The easiest way is to calculate your heart rate zones by using a basic formula.

Maximum Heart Rate = 220 - Your Age

Subtracting your age from 220 gives you a predicted max heart rate. For example, I am 42, so I subtract 42 from 220 and get 178. That number is considered my max. Now that I know my max, I can calculate my endurance or Aerobic Zone (70-80% of max), Anaerobic Zone (81-90% of max) and Anaerobic Speed Zone (91-100% of max) by multiplying your max heart rate times the percentage or zone.

178 x .70 = 124 (Aerobic Zone)

178 x .80 = 144 (Anaerobic Zone)

178 x .90 = 160 (Anaerobic Speed Zone)

EXERCISE ZONES

BEATS PER MINUTE	AGE	20	25	30	35	40	45	50	55	65	70
100%		200	195	190	185	180	175	170	165	155	150
Anaerobic Speed Zone											
90%		180	176	171	167	162	158	153	149	140	135
Anaerobic Zone											
80%		160	156	152	148	144	140	136	132	124	126
Aerobic Zone											
70%		140	137	133	130	126	123	119	116	109	105
Weight Control (Fitness / Fat burn)											
60%		120	117	114	111	108	105	102	99	93	90
Moderate Activity (Maintenance / Warm up)											
50%		100	98	95	93	90	88	85	83	78	75

Once you have your zones, you can use a heart rate monitor (chest strap) to monitor and display your zones. If you are on a treadmill or cardio piece of equipment, most of them have the ability to display your heart rate on the monitor. If you are doing cardio outside, you can download an app that will keep track while you exercise. I know I was bashing technology earlier, but here is one example where technology actually is a benefit to us. I won't get into to much detail, but know your zones and start spending 12 or more minutes in the upper zones when you work out to give you that E.P.O.C and "afterburn."

CHAPTER 8

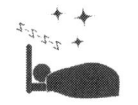

Fit Habit 3: Sleep

THIS ONE IS OF THE steps that many people disregard. They don't understand that sleep is extremely important for health and weight loss. Getting adequate sleep is necessary for your overall health and studies have shown the correlation between sleep and weight loss. Furthermore, sleep is important because of the energy it generates. If you're constantly tired, one of the things you need to look at is are you getting enough sleep at night? Now the third point, is something that I think everybody can agree on, sleep can actually attribute to more sex. Why? Because if you're tired you're going to fall asleep at night and not have the energy. So your sexual activity can increase with sleep.

The fourth reason involves two related hormones called Leptin and Ghrelin. Leptin regulates your energy balance as Ghrelin opposes it and is referred to as the "hunger hormone." When your Leptin levels drop, you start to see a slowing in your metabolism. Some studies and research have linked inadequate amount of sleep to lower levels of Leptin and higher levels of Ghrelin. More research is being done but for now just know that sleep deprivation can be a cause for increased weight gain.

How much sleep should you get? This is a bit controversial in the sense that some people can obviously function on less sleep. The general recommended amount of sleep for most people is anywhere from seven to nine hours each night. I guess that I if took a poll, it would show that most of you get less than that amount of sleep each night.

Try to avoid reading on electronic devices such as laptops, tablets and smartphones for extended periods of time before you go to sleep. These devices emit short-wavelength blue light brightly and right in your face. This exposure impairs melatonin production and interferes with your ability to fall asleep as well as with the quality of your sleep once you do nod off. My suggestion is to put down your device an hour or more before lying down to sleep.

Also, do not consume alcohol three to four hours before bedtime. If you have a glass of wine or two with dinner, great, but after that try to go three to four hours before you go to bed, and make sure you don't have anything to drink during that time period.

A final tip I suggest is before you go to bed is to take some time to visualize what you want your next day to be like. Believe it or not, that will help because you'll start thinking about that throughout the night. Make sure that what you are visualizing is a good thing. Implementing these small changes will really help with your sleep patterns.

CHAPTER 9

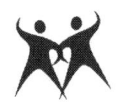

Fit Habit 4: Accountability

When it comes to being successful at reaching your goals, you need to have some accountability. Let's face it, it's hard to be consistent, Life gets in the way and before you know it you don't get your workout done. At this age in your life, you have many things going on. You may be working a full-time job, dealing with family, kids, sport activities, and then trying to fit in your own health and wellness. In my opinion, it is hard to be consistent unless you have some accountability. Also, there are no consequences for your inaction if you don't have accountability. If you're not getting it done, what's the consequence? When you have accountability built in, then it puts a little bit more added pressure to get things done.

How do you create accountability? First, you can get an accountability partner. This could be a workout buddy, a spouse, partner, or someone who has your best interest and wellbeing in mind. Make sure that whoever you choose matches the same values or follow the same habits you are trying to adhere to.

Another way is to get a coach. A good coach will not only serve as an accountability partner but as a professional who is trained to not only prescribe you the right type of exercises but to pull out the best in you. A third way would be to join an accountability group. There are lots of different groups available via social media that focus on different areas of need. I hope you will start by joining my Facebook group at

www.Facebook.com/Groups/AllAboutHealthAndFitness.

The group consists of fitness-minded members that are constantly interacting and helping people stay accountable and motivated. I highly encourage you to look for and join at least one accountability group whether it's my group or one you find on your own.

A final way to be held accountable is something that my wife and I did. For our anniversary we gave each other a FitBit to help track our daily steps, sleep, and other healthy habits.

How you keep track of your exercise is important because you want to see progression. Everything we do in life really revolves around progress, and you want to make sure that you're progressing. There are many different ways to keep track of how you're exercising, and here's where technology is now going to benefit you. If a Fitbit is not for you, you can do it the old school method by using a journal. When I first started training, I'd write down my exercises, sets and weights. The next time I came back, I knew that I wanted to increase my weight, get more reps, or achieve a specific goal. Whatever the objective was for that day, I wrote it down. Now we have lots of different apps to use to track our fitness. If you are a runner you can use Map My Run. For overall general fitness and nutrition, I like to use My Fitness Pal. Some wearable devices like a Fitbit or iWatch not only tracks your activity, but the app will track your sleep, water intake and several other health areas.

Another really unique app is Stickk.com. This site is really unique because it involves making a wager. Anytime there is money on the line people get motivated. However, this is a little different. This site allows you to set a goal and make a bet, but it's an anti-bet, meaning if you don't reach your goal, then you have to pay up. To motivate myself, I made a bet to benefit a charity that I would never support in a million years. You can make the bet to a friend or another organization to give yourself a little more motivation to reach your goal and not depart with the money. So, in my case If I didn't reach my goal and stay accountable, then I had to pay up. Looking back to my weight loss success, I attribute using this site and approach to one of the ways I got back into getting serious about my fitness after I turned 40. It really pushed me because I was so motivated to not have to pay money to a charity I personally despise. If you are looking for a fresh approach to get motivated, you could use Stickk.com to get you going.

Finally, when it comes to accountability is you need to make it public. When you put it out there publicly, for example, on social media, it holds you accountable because people you know are going to see it. Friends are going to come up to you and say, *Hey. How is it going? I know you said you were going to start training for that marathon or hey, I know that you said you wanted to lose weight, you're looking good, looks like you're sticking with your plan.*

Putting it out there publicly just makes you subconsciously realize that you have to get this done. It doesn't necessarily have to be on social media, you don't have to put it out there for everybody, but tell your significant other, tell your best friends, and tell your family about your fitness goals. Accountability is a crucial step in achieving weight loss and overall health and fitness issues. If you're serious and you want to get those results, start figuring out ways to make yourself be accountable and you'll see results.

CHAPTER 10

Fit Habit 5: Stay the Course

OVER THE YEARS, what I commonly see from former clients and people I speak with about getting fit is that they feel if they fall off the wagon that all is lost and end up totally quitting. If you take nine steps forward and eight steps back, you're still one step ahead! So don't give up, stay the course and know that you are not going to win every day. Stop being so hard on yourself and when you have a bad day, put it behind you and move on. One of my favorite mantras that I try to live by is to remember this is not a sprint but a marathon.

Bonus Step: Reward

Ok, I hope you won't mind but I have one more habit for you to start incorporating I think you're going to really like this one, and I'm calling it the bonus habit, which happens to be all about reward. Personally, I never really put much emphasis on reward earlier on with my own behaviors. I had some flawed thinking, which was if you set a goal it is just your job get it done. However, it is important that you recognize your achievement and reward yourself for reaching the goal you set for yourself. So, from now on if you are not currently rewarding yourself, I want you to start.

Reward yourself when you reach certain goals or milestones. We talked earlier about setting 12-week goals. If you reach those goals after that 12-week period, I want you to put a reward or a prize after it, and it can be something really simple, or it can be something big. It's up to you. Obviously, if you've done something amazing, and you feel like, hey, you know what, if I reach this goal, I'm going to go out and buy myself a brand new wardrobe. I'm going to spend a couple hundred bucks, or I'm going to buy myself a new purse, or I'm going to go get myself a new watch. Whatever it is, reward yourself. Life is meant to be fun, and I think you should enjoy it.

I'm not one of those coaches who think it's all work and no play. I enjoy going out to a nice dinner. I enjoy having a glass of wine. I enjoy eating queso. Yeah, you heard me, I enjoy it. And you should, too. So if you work really hard, and you reach some milestone, you reach a goal, it's okay to reward yourself. Go out and enjoy and don't worry about it. Indulge all you want, but get back to those healthy habits before you lose everything you worked so hard for!

CHAPTER 11

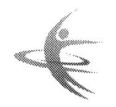

What's Next?

DON'T MAKE THIS MISTAKE of reading all the way through this book, picking up some great knowledge, coming up with your "why," and NOT taking action. The purpose behind this book is for you to understand that it's not difficult to lose weight and get fit. You don't need a crazy hyped up workout plan to get results.

This is more about just shifting mindsets, implementing simple strategies, and ultimately taking action. Whenever I finish reading a book, I like to have a step-by-step plan to follow, so I've provided one for you.

Step One

Make the commitment that you are going to change, that you are going to take action daily. It doesn't have to be perfect, but you have to start. Every day, I want you to do something that's going to improve your health and improve your life. Strive to improve your health by 1% every day.

Step Two

Set your 12-week S.M.A.R.T. goal. If you need to, go back and re-read the section that talks about the 12-week year and S.M.A.R.T. and set your goals today. Once you have those goals set, make them public. It doesn't have to be to everyone on social media, but tell a spouse, a friend, or send it to me in an email at dave@davemcgarry.com with the subject line *Re: My SMART GOALS.*

Step Three

Get an accountability partner, such as a friend or a significant other. If you need one, reach out to me and I'll be your accountability partner and your coach. Also, if you need a workout partner, find one.

Step Four

Start implementing HIIT workouts in your exercise routine. You need to get at least three to four high intensity interval training sessions per week in your schedule if you want to accelerate your results. Doing this is going to allow your body to burn calories 12-36 hours after your workout. Plus, typically you will be pushing yourself harder during these types of workouts so you will probably burn more during the workout then you would doing something else.

Step Five

Plan out your nutrition. Think about what you're going to eat for the week on Sundays. That means you have an idea and plan for Monday, Tuesday, Wednesday, Thursday, Friday, and Saturday. If you want to plan one cheat day per week, then go ahead and do that. A bonus tip about the cheat day is to only have one every other week. Go a full seven days then have a cheat day and then another seven days. This pushes you through the weekend days that for some people are the worst days when it comes to their nutritional habits.

Step Six

Start tracking your workouts, at least initially, so you can find out whether or not you're making progress. Always change up the amount of weight and reps you do in each workout. A sure way to waste your time and not see progress is to do the same exercises, reps, and weights every time you workout. The reason is because the body needs to be stimulated differently. It will adapt to whatever demand you put on it so by doing the same routine over and over, your body will eventually be used to the stimulus and stop responding to it in a positive way. The other bonus to tracking your workouts is when you look back you have a written document record of your progress. Trust me, you will be amazed at where you started!

Implement these six steps now. Don't delay! I hope this book will help you feel motivated to take action and start implementing change into your life right away!

Case Study: How I Lost 25 lbs.

I've told you about my struggles and the low point in my fitness journey. I am using this as a case study and example of the step-by-step process I used myself, and the process I use with all my clients to get results. You will see that most of what I wrote about in this book I implemented into my own life. I originally had this in the beginning of the book but I rearranged it to place it here so maybe you will understand the concepts I preach and coach to my clients. As you will see I implemented them into my weight loss journey and I hope it helps you with your mission!

About a year before I turned 40, I was at my heaviest weight at 217 lbs. and I thought that I was in shape! A typical workout for me would be to do 30 minutes on the elliptical, do some weight lifting here and there, and eat decently. My workouts had become routine and I was no longer getting outside my comfort zone while working out.

I realized that this potentially is midlife for me and I had to ask myself if I wanted to continue down a slow path of deteriorating health or did I want to get in the best shape of my life. This was the second turning point for me. When my father passed away, I made a decision then to make my health a priority, but I had once again become complacent with my fitness. Again, I decided it was time to make a change!

Now that I had made a decision to change, I took the first step that I recommend all my clients to do and set a S.M.A.R.T goal. The S.M.A.R.T goal I set for myself was to lose 10 pounds in 90 days. The goal weight was to be at

207 by mid April. Once I reached that first goal I set another S.M.A.R.T goal, which was another 10 pounds. Again 90 days later, I hit my goal and was now weighing in at 192 lbs. down from where I was six months earlier. Initially 20 lbs. was what I wanted to accomplish as the end result but as I started to lose weight and feel great again I decided why stop there so I set another goal to reach 193. A weight I have not weighed since my college days. This required a little more effort and discipline but around 9 months into the journey I hit 192. Now, I know a lot of people want to lose at a faster rate, but I did it in nine months, and I did it mainly by setting safe, small goals of 10 lbs. at a time, and then setting new goals once I reached my initial goal that I set.

Now that's not all I did. I wish it was that simple but I actually had to get more disciplined and create some daily habits. I know a lot of people think you have to get crazy and live at the gym to see significant weight loss but that is far from the truth. Actually if you spend 1 hour a day working out that is only 4 % of your day so that still leaves 96% of your day doing other things like getting enough sleep, eating right and drinking enough water. So, the first thing I did was I assessed my nutritional habits. There were things I was eating I feel contributed to me gaining weight; foods like high starchy carbs type, sugars, and foods higher in unhealthy fat such as fast food, and regular ground beef. Also, from my background in Exercise Science and studying of nutrition I knew that my protein intake was not nearly as high as it should be so I made an effort to supplement my protein everyday. Since my schedule is pretty busy with family and work I knew the best way for me to supplement my protein was to have a protein shake every morning. I also started preparing my weekly meals every Sunday, and along with eating more protein I made an effort to eat less starchy carbs. You know the ones like pasta, bread and rice! Finally, my workouts changed. Instead of getting up and doing 30 minutes on the elliptical just to say I got my thirty minutes in, I started doing high intensity interval training. Sessions ranged from 30 minutes to an hour, 2-3 times a week. Regardless of the length of the workout, the big difference was the fact I was getting my heart rate up and achieving

EPOC. This allowed my body to burn calories longer and ultimately accelerate fat loss.

So, when I say that I didn't do anything crazy, I mean it. All I did was set S.M.A.R.T. goals, change my workout routine by doing HIIT workouts and got my mindset right about why I wanted my health and fitness levels to be! Pretty simple and you can do the same!

CHAPTER 12

My Fit Over 40 Inspiration

I WANT TO LEAVE YOU some inspiration to take the Fit Over 40 Challenge by sharing a couple of my role models.

My Grandfather

My grandfather lived to the age of 97. I can remember as a kid growing up my grandfather would follow a routine. Every day he walked for 30 minutes to an hour. He did sit-ups and pushups and kept his mind active by reading the paper. He ate an apple every day and drank a glass of wine at dinner at night. When he got older (mid 70's), he had worn out the cartilage in his knee and shoulder so he swam several times a week in the therapeutic pool. I joked with him and said we need to get you to set the Guinness Book of World Records for the amount of laps someone your age swims at a time. That always made him chuckle! Not only did he swim, but also he was very active and functional well into his 90's. If he were here to tell you himself, he would say it was due to his fitness routine and healthy lifestyle. He was a true inspiration to me!

My Mother

My mother is now is in her mid 70's. A few years ago, we went to Disney with the kids and did one of those marathon days walking the park from dawn until almost midnight and my mom was right there with us stride for stride. She tells me how impressed members of her gym are with her as she takes all the group exercise classes with women half her age. She is probably in better shape than most 40-year-olds today.

I know that it can be done, and those are just a couple of personal examples. If you did a Google search on "inspirational stories of fit people over 40," you would find countless examples of people who have done remarkable feats.

Do yourself a favor and don't let your age be a factor in you getting into the best shape of your life because I know you can be fit at any age. Maybe you have never really thought about how your life can affect others around you. My dad never really thought his health issues affected me or really had me concerned. You need to think differently about really why you want to be fit and live a healthy active lifestyle. There will be roadblocks and obstacles along the way, but your "why" is going to push you through it. When you establish a strong enough "why," I can guarantee you that change will occur!

CHAPTER 13

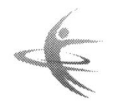

Take the Challenge

IF YOU HAVE MADE IT this far, I know you are serious about taking control of your life and making being fit a priority. I have said this book is not like a typical fitness book that offers up a new workout plan or diet for you to follow, but more of a road map to get you started on seeing results. However, as with anything you can't just study and learn, you need to start taking action and implement. So, I am going to ask you to take the *Fit Over 40 Challenge*. The challenge is all about getting you started and supporting you during your first six weeks.

Let me be clear and set expectations with you. Not everyone is going to see major transformations when it comes to weight loss. For some, this six-week challenge will be challenging just by doing something small every day to get you moving in the right direction. For others, this will be a good jump-start to getting you back on track and moving in the right direction again. I said this earlier and I will say it again, I am not here to present some flash and sizzle marketing hype just to sell books. Real long-term transformation takes time.

For legal purposes I have to post this disclaimer and note:

Disclaimer: Not all programs are appropriate for everyone. Consult your doctor before starting this program. This manual and program are not intended as medical advice and do not take the place of medical advice or treatment from your doctor. The author shall not be held liable or responsible for any misuse of this information or any loss, damage, injury caused or alleged to be caused directly or indirectly by any of use of this information or these workouts. This information is not intended to diagnose, treat, cure or prevent any disease or illness.

Note: Due to recent statements from the FTC, it is required that we identify what a "typical" result is. The harsh truth is that most people never do anything with the products they buy, so most of the time, their typical results are zero. You are the main element of your success! Our clients have lost hundreds of pounds of fat, increased lean muscle and increased their performance using this system. The people that show even greater success worked hard, and earned their results. As with any exercise program, obtain the consent of your doctor before the initiation of any physical training program.

For further information and additional services, including consulting and speaking engagements, please see our website:

www.fitover40challenge.com.

CHAPTER 14

The Fit Over 40 Challenge Begins

Congratulations on making it this far! It is time to start moving and join the challenge to get fit and healthy at 40 and above!

This challenge is broken into two parts: The Warm-up and the weekly assignments for the next six weeks. I know you got this!!

Warm-up

20-30 seconds of running in place

20-30 seconds of running in place "butt-kicks"

20-30 seconds of hands behind head "high-knees"

20-30 seconds of fake "jump-rope"

10 arm circles to the front

10 arm circles to the back

10 leg swings each leg (forward and backward and side to side)

REPEAT ONCE MORE - Looking for 3 - 5 minute warm-up

6-Week Program

Week #1

Goal Setting – 12-week S.M.A.R.T. goal - Make yourself accountable by posting to Facebook.com/Groups/AllAboutHealthAndFitness or find an accountability partner.

Change One Nutritional Bad Habit – If you would like to get a list of healthy food options and get a "jump start," you can get started on the "7 Day Fat Loss Challenge by going to the at

www.FitOver40Challenge.com/FatLoss

Let's Get Started

Warm-up (See above)

Exercises Week #1 - "The Dirty 30"

- 30 Push-ups (rest if you need to but get it done)
- 30 Alternating reverse lunges with hands on head (15 for each leg)
- 30 Jump Squats
- 30 Burpees

I want you to do this workout 3 times this week. It can be Monday/Wednesday/Friday or Tuesday/Thursday/ Saturday

On the off days, make sure you stretch and get some form of cardio in for at least 20 minutes. My suggestion on the off day cardio is to incorporate some interval training such as sprints or hill climbs to get the heart rate elevated.

Week #2

On day one, revisit goals and set intentions for the week.

Add 1-2 more changes in habits (for example, replace soda or diet soda with water; add one healthier food option while eliminating a processed food)

Exercises Week #2 - "Up The Ladder, Down The Ladder"

- 5 Close Grip Push-ups
- 10 Mountain Climbers
- 15 Reverse Crunches
- 20 Bicycle kicks (abs)
- 25 Toe Touches (feet in the air)
- 30 Squats
- 35 Fake jump ropes
- 40 Alternating forward lunges with hands behind head (20 each side) then go in reverse back to 35, 30, 25, etc.

Rest 90 seconds when you have gone up and down the ladder, then repeat one more time!

I want you to do this workout three times this week. It can be Monday/Wednesday/Friday or Tuesday/Thursday/ Saturday

On the off days, make sure you stretch and get some form of cardio in for at least 20 minutes.

Week # 3

Set intentions for this week and revisit goals.

Add a fitness habit to the 3-4 changes you have already made (for example, park your car further away from a building and walk; take the stairs instead of riding the elevator).

Exercises Week #3 - "Quadzilla"

- 10 Squats
- 10 Right leg reverse lunges
- 10 Right leg forward lunges
- 10 Left leg reverse lunges
- 10 left leg forward lunges
- 10 Burpees (add pushup for advanced move)
- 10 Jump Squats

Rest 1 minute, then repeat 3 more times!

I want you to do this workout 3 times this week. It can be Monday/Wednesday/Friday or Tuesday/Thursday/ Saturday

Week # 4

Revisit goals and set intentions for the week.

Either add to fitness habits or really focus in on the one or two that will make a bigger impact for your weight loss goals (for example, cut out processed foods and refined sugar foods).

Exercises Week #4 - "Go off the Grid"

We are going to incorporate a little outdoor atmosphere into the mix.

- 20 seconds of all out "run like you stole something" running, immediately followed by 10 squats with hands behind hand and finishing with 10 push-ups.
- Rest 40 seconds then repeat 6 more times for a total of 7 "all-out" sprints.
- I want you to do this workout 3 times this week. It can either be

Monday/Wednesday/Friday or
Tuesday/Thursday/ Saturday

Week # 5

Revisit goals and set intentions at the beginning of the week.

Again, focus in on the one or two fitness habits that are going to make the most difference for you. It may be to up the intensity of the exercises or to add another day or two to being physically active

Exercises Week #5 - "Random Pick"

Pick three of the exercise routines from weeks one through four and do one Monday, another Wednesday, and the third Friday.

If you are doing Tuesday/Thursday/Saturday, do the same thing I suggested for the Monday/Wednesday/Friday pattern.

Week # 6

Set intentions and revisit goals one more time.

Make this week your best week and adhere to all the fitness habits that you changed throughout the first 5 weeks.

Exercises Week #6 - "Choose Again But Add Something"

I want you to do the same thing you did for week 5, but I am adding an additional cardio workout for you to do at the gym. If you do not have a current gym membership, then do the outside cardio workout twice this week. You will be working out 4 times this week. If you still have your chain gym membership and you use the cardio machines, or if you have an elliptical or treadmill at home, or if you are visiting a hotel, here is a good workout to do that is way more effective than "steady-state cardio" and it's faster. This can be done any piece of equipment.

Note: Level 1-10 is a "perceived level of difficulty" meaning level 1 is like sitting on a couch, level 4-6 is challenging but doable, and level 10 is where you feel miserable.

This is not what the treadmill or elliptical speed or level is – this is what YOU perceive to be for YOUR BODY.

Person A might think that a level 5 for her is running at a speed of 6.7 on the treadmill while person B who is out of shape might think that level 5 for her is simply walking.

Minute 0-2 – level 5 (for you)

Minute 2-3 – level 6

Minute 3-4 – level 7

Minute 4-5 – level 8

Minute 5-6 – level 9

Minute 6-7 – level 6

Minute 7-8 – level 7

Minute 8-9 – level 8

Minute 9-10 – level 9

Minute 10-11 – level 6

Minute 11-12 – level 7

Minute 12-13 – level 8

Minute 13-14 – level 9

Minute 14-15 – level 6

Minute 15-16 – level 7

Minute 16-17 – level 8

Minute 17-18 – level 9

Minute 18-19 – level 10 * this is the all out minute (empty the tank)

Minute 19-23 – cool down back at level 5 (recover and stretch)

Congratulations, you completed the six-week challenge! Don't forget to celebrate your win by sharing on social media or telling someone who cares about you. Reward yourself by going out to a nice dinner or buying some new clothes. Life is meant to be enjoyed and lived.

Remember, health and fitness is a marathon and not a sprint. You are going to have periods of time where it all just seems to click and you feel like you are 20 again. Then there will be times that you feel tired and your efforts don't seem to be paying off. Stay the course and just keep grinding! You've got this!

P.S. If you found this book to be helpful and you feel it would benefit someone, please let them know about it. My goal is to help as many people as I possibly can and a 5-star review on Amazon will allow me to hopefully get this into the hands of others who might benefit from it so I would appreciate the review!

In health,
Coach Dave
www.FitOver40Challenge.com

Message From David

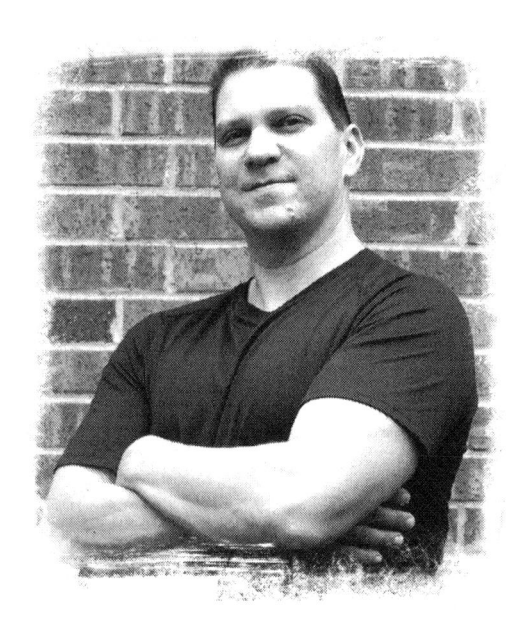

I want to congratulate you for making a decision to take control of your life and get healthy and fit.

My personal mission is to help educate, inspire, and guide you on becoming fit over 40 and beyond so you can live an extraordinary life by using the principles and strategies I lay out in the book.

I know that there are things you might still have questions about and may need more instruction, so I have put together a resources page on my website just for those of you who have purchased the book. For additional tips, videos, and more, visit:

www.FitOver40Challenge.com/BookResources

Made in the USA
Charleston, SC
23 February 2017